AROMA INHALATION THERAPY

A Complete Guide On Awakening The Senses Of Tranquility And Embracing Wellness Through Scents

WALTER ZYAIRE

© [Walter Zyaire] [2024]. All rights reserved.

No part of this book may be reproduced, stored in a retrieval system, or transmitted in any form or by any means, electronic, mechanical, photocopying, recording, or otherwise, without the express written permission of the author, with the exception of small extracts in critical reviews or articles.

DISCLAIMER

The information in this book is intended only for general informational purposes; it should not be used in lieu of professional advice or medical care. Since the author is not licensed to practice therapy, the information offered should not be used in place of the expertise, judgment, or guidance of qualified mental health or medical professionals. Readers are encouraged to consult therapists, medical specialists, or other qualified authorities regarding their particular situation and needs. The publisher and author disclaim all liability for any actions or decisions taken by readers based on the information in this book. Results may vary from person to person and this book's approaches, procedures, and strategies may not be suitable in all circumstances. Considering unique situations and consulting a qualified expert are essential when choosing the right course of action. Neither the publisher nor the author recommend or guarantee the efficacy of any therapy or treatment that is indicated in this book. Because the information is based on the author's research and understanding at the time of publishing, it could not reflect the most recent developments or practices in the treatment area. The publisher and the author both disclaim all liability for the accuracy, completeness, or use of the material in this book. Readers bear full responsibility for the decisions and actions they choose in light of the information presented in this book.

TABLE OF CONTENTS

ABOUT THIS BOOK

"Aroma Inhalation Therapy" is an extensive manual that explores the intriguing realm of aromatherapy and its significant influence on overall health. This book is significant because it gives readers a comprehensive understanding of aroma inhalation therapy and a useful tool for utilizing essential oils for better physical, mental, and emotional well-being.

The book begins with a thoughtful introduction that establishes the framework for the rest of the discussion of aromatherapy. The first few chapters concentrate on laying the groundwork for aromatherapy, including key concepts, historical viewpoints, and the characteristics of essential oils. This firm foundation lays the groundwork for a more thorough comprehension of fragrance inhalation therapy, clarifying its advantages, drawbacks, and modes of action.

After that, readers are taken through the wide range of essential oils and their uses, learning about popular oils, key safety precautions, and mixing methods.

With the use of methods and technologies like roll-ons, vaporizers, inhalers, and diffusers, readers may incorporate fragrance inhalation into their everyday routines with ease.

The book's concentration on particular uses of fragrance inhalation therapy is one of its strong points. Targeted advice on employing scents to address common wellness concerns is provided in the chapters on energy, focus, sleep, relaxation, and stress alleviation. The investigation of scents for mental health emphasizes how adaptable aromatherapy is even more.

The book also offers helpful guidance on using scent inhalation in daily life, going beyond theory. Readers discover how to easily integrate aromatherapy into their daily routines, whether at home, at work, or through portable solutions.

A special chapter devoted to research and studies highlights the scientific basis of fragrance inhalation therapy, offering evidence-based methods and outlining potential future developments in the field. Responsible handling of cautions and contraindications guarantees that readers are aware of any possible hazards, including drug interactions, allergies, and sensitivities.

 A thorough tutorial on making custom fragrance blends is included at the end of the book, enabling readers to customize aromatherapy to suit their tastes and requirements. The book's usefulness as a practical manual for fragrance inhalation therapy is further demonstrated by the case studies that illustrate how these concepts are applied in real-world settings. All things considered, "Aroma Inhalation Therapy" is an essential tool for beginners as well as experts, providing a comprehensive and knowledgeable approach to the healing potential of aromatherapy.

CHAPTER ONE

OVERVIEW OF AROMA INHALATION THERAPY

THE AROMA INHALATION THERAPY

Aromatherapy, also known as aroma inhalation therapy, is a holistic healing technique that improves mental, emotional, and physical well-being by utilizing the therapeutic qualities of aromatic molecules. This treatment's main idea is inhaling aromatic plant extracts, or essential oils, which come from a variety of plant components, including flowers, leaves, stems, and roots. It is thought that these concentrated aromatic compounds have significant impacts on mood, relaxation, and general wellness in humans.

The origins of aromatherapy can be traced back hundreds of years, to the periods of ancient Egypt, China, and India. These societies adopted fragrances into daily life, medical procedures, and religious ceremonies after realizing the smells' powerful therapeutic abilities. To improve wellness, aromatherapy is now a widely used alternative therapy that can be used either alone or in conjunction with traditional medicine.

Knowing the wide variety of essential oils that are accessible, each with distinct qualities and therapeutic advantages is one of the most important things to know about Aroma Inhalation Therapy.

By carefully extracting these oils using techniques like distillation or cold pressing, the volatile components that give them their unique smells and therapeutic qualities are preserved. Among the essential oils frequently used in aromatherapy are lavender, eucalyptus, peppermint, and chamomile. Each oil has a unique set of uses and physiological effects.

AROMAS' SIGNIFICANCE TO WELL-BEING

The powerful effects that smell can have on the body and mind of a person made them important for overall well-being.

The foundation of aromatherapy is the idea that particular smells have the power to elicit strong feelings, bring back memories, and affect one's general state of mind. The limbic system, which is important for emotions, memories, and bodily processes, is closely linked to the olfactory system, which is in charge of smell.

Aromas can elicit a multitude of feelings, ranging from alertness and renewal to calmness and relaxation. This emotional and psychological impact is used in the context of well-being to reduce stress, anxiety, and other emotional dysregulation.

Calming essential oils like lavender and chamomile are frequently used to create a peaceful environment that encourages relaxation and aids with stress management.

Moreover, there are physiological advantages linked to inhaling specific scents. For instance, eucalyptus oil is well-known for its respiratory advantages, as it facilitates easier breathing by clearing nasal passages.

Because peppermint oil has energizing qualities that promote alertness and mental clarity, it is frequently utilized. It is thought that these aromatic chemicals have molecular interactions with the body, affecting things like blood pressure, hormone balance, and heart rate.

Scents have a significant impact on mental and physical health because they stimulate the senses, arouse feelings, and engage the senses. With its deep historical origins and contemporary uses, Aroma Inhalation Therapy provides a comprehensive method of enhancing health and well-being by carefully utilizing the fragrant treasures of nature.

CHAPTER TWO

THE BASICS OF AROMATHERAPY

HISTORICAL VIEWS

With its roots in antiquity, aromatherapy has a rich historical background spanning numerous nations and civilizations. Aromatherapy has its roots in the ancient world, specifically in Egypt, where essential oils were utilized in religious rituals, medicine, and even the mummification process. The holistic approach that is embodied by aromatherapy was first recognized by the Greeks and Romans, who also welcomed fragrant substances for their healing properties.

The middle Ages saw a continuing advancement in the understanding of essential oils as botanical research and distillation methods were improved. The Renaissance saw a rise in interest in aromatic compounds and herbal medicines, which aided in the creation of aromatherapy. The term "aromatherapy" was first used in the 20th century by the French chemist René-Maurice Gattefossé, who conducted a thorough investigation into the therapeutic qualities of essential oils, especially after he witnessed how well they worked for burn patients.

THE FUNDAMENTALS OF AROMATHERAPY

The basis of aromatherapy is the idea that aromatic substances that are taken from plants and referred to as essential oils have healing qualities that can enhance mental, emotional, and physical health. The practice is based on the idea that these volatile substances interact with the body's chemistry to promote harmony and balance when applied or inhaled. A fundamental idea is the holistic approach, which takes into account the full person in addition to treating certain symptoms.

Essential oils are hand-picked for their medicinal properties and distinct chemical compositions. The application technique—diffusion, topical usage, or inhalation—is selected to maximize the absorption of these powerful oils.

Aromatherapy acknowledges the importance of emotional and psychological states in general health, emphasizing the connection between the mind and body.

PROPERTIES OF ESSENTIAL OILS

The foundation of aromatherapy is concentrated hydrophobic liquids called essential oils that contain plant-based volatile scent components. The various chemical compositions of essential oils, which include terpenes, aldehydes, ketones, and phenols, give birth to their varied qualities. Every essential oil has a unique profile that adds to its medicinal qualities.

For example, lavender is often used for relaxation and stress treatment due to its well-known relaxing and soothing qualities. Tea tree oil is used for its purifying and cleansing properties because of its strong antibacterial properties. Peppermint is preferred for its energizing and cooling properties, while eucalyptus is praised for its respiratory advantages.

Comprehending the distinct characteristics of every essential oil is crucial for crafting harmonious mixtures that address a range of health issues. Aromatherapists utilize a thorough evaluation of elements such as chemical composition, extraction techniques, and botanical origin to fully utilize these natural extracts in supporting overall health.

CHAPTER THREE

AN EXPLANATION OF AROMA INHALATION THERAPY

COMPREHENDING AROMA INHALATION

Aromatherapy, sometimes referred to as aroma inhalation therapy, is a holistic treatment technique that uses fragrant plant extracts, also called essential oils, to support mental, emotional, and physical health. The ability to use fragrance to elicit therapeutic effects is the basic idea underlying aroma inhalation. This age-old custom has its origins in the usage of fragrant materials to promote spiritual experiences and treat medical ailments in several ancient civilizations.

MECHANISMS OF ACTION

Aroma inhalation treatment is based on complex mechanisms of action that encompass both physiological and psychological responses. Volatile molecules from essential oils when breathed enter the nasal cavity, where olfactory receptors identify and send signals to the limbic system, a sophisticated network of brain structures linked to memory and emotions. The brain and olfactory system are directly connected, which explains why breathing in aromas can have a strong emotional impact and affect mood.

The inhaled chemicals may also interact with the respiratory system physiologically. The aromatic molecules can have a calming or energizing effect on people's respiratory tracts when they breathe them in. Certain essential oils have antibacterial qualities that could aid in the treatment of allergies or respiratory infections, enhancing respiratory health.

ADVANTAGES

Aroma inhalation treatment has a plethora of potential advantages for anyone looking for safe, all-natural solutions for a range of health issues. The principal benefit lies in its capacity to promote relaxation and mitigate stress.

Some essential oils are well known for their ability to induce calmness and help with sleep difficulties. Examples of these oils are lavender and chamomile.

Aroma inhalation can also be used to improve focus and cognitive performance. The stimulating qualities of essential oils, such as those found in peppermint and rosemary can enhance mental clarity and attention. The application of certain essential oils has been acknowledged for its ability to mitigate headaches and migraines due to their analgesic and anti-inflammatory characteristics.

RESTRICTIONS

Even though fragrance inhalation treatment has grown in popularity and has shown promising results, it is important to recognize its limitations. First of all, different people react differently to aromatherapy, so what works for one person could not have the same effect on another. Essential oils' effectiveness is a matter of opinion that is impacted by a variety of variables, including sensitivities, health issues, and personal preferences.

Furthermore, even while fragrance inhalation can support traditional medical procedures, it shouldn't be used in place of expert medical guidance. Serious medical disorders need to be properly diagnosed and treated by licensed medical practitioners. Aroma inhalation therapy is generally safe when used as directed; nevertheless, misuse or overuse of particular essential oils can cause negative effects, so moderation and caution are key.

Aroma inhalation therapy is a comprehensive strategy that harnesses the therapeutic and physiological effects of scent. For those looking to include this practice in their wellness regimens, it is essential to comprehend its processes of action, potential benefits, and restrictions. To ensure safe and successful integration into one's overall health plan, it is advisable to consult with healthcare specialists as with any complementary therapy.

CHAPTER FOUR

APPLICATIONS OF ESSENTIAL OILS
FREQUENTLY USED ESSENTIAL OILS

Essential oils are becoming more and more well-known due to their many uses and medicinal qualities. Lavender oil is one of the most popular essential oils, valued for its relaxing and comforting properties. It is frequently used in aromatherapy to encourage calmness and reduce tension. Tea tree oil is another popular essential oil that is used frequently because of its antifungal and antibacterial qualities. Tea tree oil is frequently used in skincare products and treatments for several types of skin ailments. Because of its well-known stimulating and cooling aroma, peppermint oil is frequently used in aromatherapy and as a home treatment for headaches.

Because of its well-known respiratory advantages, eucalyptus oil is widely utilized in steam inhalations as a congestion reliever. The citrus fruit that yields lemon oil is prized for its invigorating and stimulating scent. It is frequently utilized in diffusers and cleaning supplies to produce a clean, energizing atmosphere. Furthermore, chamomile oil, which is derived from chamomile flowers, is prized for its relaxing qualities and is frequently used in aromatherapy and cosmetic products to encourage calmness.

BLENDING METHODS

The skill of blending essential oils entails mixing various oils to produce a scent that is harmonic and well-balanced or to intensify particular therapeutic properties. Using top, middle, and base notes is a typical blending method.

The top notes provide a freshness boost and are the first smells that are detected. Base notes give depth and stability to the overall perfume, while middle notes bring richness and body to the combination. It takes trial and error with ratios and careful consideration of the desired result—be it energy, relaxation, or a particular therapeutic effect—to create a well-balanced combination.

It's critical to take into account each oil's chemical components and any potential synergies or contraindications. Certain oils blend well together, while others might not be good for blending.

The blending process can be improved by experimenting with small amounts and recording the combinations. Furthermore, since it affects how long the smell of the mix lasts, it is vital to comprehend the volatility of certain oils.

GUIDELINES FOR SAFETY

While utilizing essential oils has many advantages, it's important to put safety first. The right dilution is crucial since undiluted essential oils can irritate or sensitize the skin. Diluting essential oils for topical use involves the use of carrier oils, like jojoba or coconut oil.

Following precise dilution ratios is advised, particularly when applying oils to young people or people with sensitive skin.

 Certain people with specific medical issues or those who are pregnant may be in danger from certain essential oils. In such circumstances, it is advisable to look up the contraindications of particular oils and speak with a healthcare provider. Since heat and sunshine can gradually deteriorate the quality of essential oils, proper storage is also crucial. Finally, it's important to utilize essential oils sparingly since overusing them—even when they're well-diluted—can have negative effects. All things considered, using essential oils safely and enjoyingly can be achieved by exercising caution and being aware of personal sensitivities.

CHAPTER FIVE

INSTRUMENTS AND METHODS

DIFFUSERS AND VAPORIZERS

Aromatherapy is a popular technique that uses fragrant essential oils to support mental and physical health. Diffusers and vaporizers are common instruments for aromatherapy. By releasing essential oils into the atmosphere, these gadgets enable users to breathe in healing aromas. There are many different kinds of diffusers, such as evaporative, nebulizing, and ultrasonic diffusers.

Nebulizing diffusers break down the oils into a fine mist without using water, whereas ultrasonic diffusers use water to disseminate a fine mist of essential oil and water into the air. A fan is used in evaporative diffusers to force air through a pad or filter that holds essential oils, dispersing the aroma throughout the room. Conversely, vaporizers usually use heat to cause the volatile components of essential oils to be released into the atmosphere. Diffusers and vaporizers offer a practical and efficient means of reaping the advantages of aromatherapy, which include heightened mood, reduced tension, and relaxation.

ROLL-ONS AND INHALERS

Roll-ons and inhalers are lightweight, easily handled devices that provide a more focused application of aromatherapy. Inhalers sometimes referred to as nose inhalers or personal inhalers, are made of a little tube with a cotton wick soaked in essential oils inside of it. Users can enjoy unobtrusive aromatherapy while on the go by just inhaling the scent through their noses. Inhalers are frequently utilized for targeted uses, like relieving headaches, improving focus, or reducing congestion. Conversely, roll-ons are applicators that have a mixture of essential oils diluted with a carrier oil in them. The roll-on can be immediately applied to the skin, wrists, temples, or other pulse spots by the user. This technique enables topical application, offering the advantages of skin absorption and aromatherapy in tandem. If you're looking for a more specialized and individualized approach to aromatherapy, roll-ons, and inhalers are handy solutions that let you discreetly and conveniently address certain difficulties or concerns.

Do-it-yourself (DIY) aroma inhalation techniques give people the freedom to customize aromatherapy treatments to suit their requirements and tastes. Using essential oils and a basin of hot water is one well-liked do-it-yourself technique. A few drops of the essential oils of their choice are added to hot water by users, resulting in a steam that releases the aromatic molecules into the atmosphere. After that, they can breathe in the steam for a comforting and healing experience.

Making homemade inhaler mixes by mixing essential oils with carrier oil, and then filling a blank inhaler tube with the combination, is another do-it-yourself option. This enables people to customize the scent to their preferences and target particular wellness objectives.

Additionally, a quick and adaptable approach to enjoy aromatherapy throughout the house is to use essential oils on a cloth sachet or in a bowl of potpourri. With the help of DIY scent inhalation techniques, people can experiment with various essential oil mixtures to create a unique and pleasurable sensory experience that fits their tastes and wellness objectives.

CHAPTEER SIX

AROMATHERAPY TO DE-STRESS AND PROMOTE RELAXATION

AROMATHERAPY & RELAXING SCENTS

One of the most well-known scents for its relaxing qualities is lavender. Aromatherapy plays a big part in encouraging relaxation and stress reduction. Because of its calming properties for both the body and mind, lavender has been utilized for ages. Lavender scents are said to lessen anxiety and encourage serenity. According to research, breathing in lavender essential oil has a calming effect on the nervous system and promotes relaxation. To create a calm atmosphere that promotes relaxation, many people include lavender in their daily routines through essential oils, candles, or sachets.

Apart from lavender, several other soothing aromas aid in relieving stress. Aromas with calming properties, such as jasmine, bergamot, and chamomile, are well known. These scents function by altering the brain's emotional centers and inducing a relaxing response through interactions with the olfactory system. These soothing aromas can be applied topically with massage oils or diffused into the air to create a peaceful environment that eases tension and encourages relaxation.

METHODS FOR RELAXATION

Aside from scents, several methods support stress relief and relaxation. An essential technique for lowering tension and calming the nervous system is deep breathing. To induce physical and mental calm, progressive muscle relaxation entails methodically tensing and then relaxing various muscle groups. Through the practice of mindfulness and meditation, people can cultivate a sense of peace by learning to concentrate on the here and now.

The practice of aromatherapy is using essential oils to improve both physical and mental health.

Aromatherapy diffusers, inhalers, and massage oils are popular devices for administering scents. An opulent and successful method of relaxing might also be taking a warm bath scented with relaxing aromas. A holistic approach to stress management is created when aromatherapy is combined with other relaxation techniques, addressing both the physical and emotional elements of tension.

USING AROMATHERAPY TO MANAGE STRESS

By utilizing the healing qualities of different fragrances, aromatherapy is a potent technique for stress management. Aromas have the power to affect stress levels and mood because of the olfactory system, which is intimately connected to the brain's emotional regions. Plants are used to extract essential oils, which are volatile substances that have the power to elicit particular emotions.

Aromatherapy can be incorporated into daily routines by topical treatments like massage oils or balms, or by using diffusers, which release essential oils into the air. Essential oils that are popular for alleviating stress include frankincense, eucalyptus, lavender, and chamomile. Tailoring aromatherapy mixes to individual preferences enables people to customize their approach to managing stress.

It's important to remember that, even while aromatherapy can be a useful tool in stress reduction; it functions best when combined with other comprehensive stress management techniques. The synergistic effect of combining aromatherapy with other relaxation methods, lifestyle changes, and self-care routines improves general well-being. Individual reactions to smells can differ, as with any therapeutic method, so it's best to experiment and find the scents that work best for you to de-stress and unwind.

CHAPTER SEVEN

FRAGRANCES FOR VIGOR AND CONCENTRATION

CITRUS AND ENERGIZING AROMAS

Aromas that are energizing and citrus-based are essential for improving concentration and vitality. Citrus fruit smells, which include lemon, orange, and grapefruit, are known to excite the senses and increase alertness. These aromas are zesty and invigorating. These smells can assist generate a revitalizing atmosphere and are known to have an instantaneous effect on mood. Citrus scents are said to be energizing because they trigger the production of neurotransmitters like serotonin, which elevates mood and increases vitality.

INCREASING FOCUS

Increasing focus is a typical objective for people looking to improve their cognitive function and productivity. Aromas, especially those that have mental-stirring qualities, can be quite helpful in accomplishing this goal. Some essential oils, like eucalyptus and peppermint, are well known for their capacity to increase mental clarity and attention. It's thought that breathing in these energizing aromas improves blood flow to the brain, which enhances cognitive performance and maintains concentration. Adding these scents to one's surroundings—through diffusers or topically—can help create an environment that is better suited for focus.

TAKING ON FATIGUE

Aromas might be useful partners in the fight against weariness. Physical or mental exhaustion can seriously impair well-being and productivity. Aromatherapy with essential oils such as peppermint, lavender, and rosemary has demonstrated the potential to reduce fatigue and encourage a refreshed state of mind. These scents are thought to offer energizing qualities that, by improving circulation, lowering stress levels, and energizing the body and mind, can aid in the fight against fatigue. Setting up a room filled with these energizing aromas can be a healthy, all-natural way to fight exhaustion and provide a much-needed energy boost.

The potent influence that smells have on our senses is the foundation for the application of aromas for attention and energy. Fragrances with citrus and energizing properties help to increase alertness, improve focus, and fight fatigue. Whether it's from the energizing qualities of citrus fruits or the invigorating qualities of essential oils, introducing these scents into everyday spaces can foster a more alert and concentrated state of mind, enhancing general well-being and efficiency.

CHAPTER EIGHT

SLEEPING WITH AN AROMATHERAPY INHALATION

CALM AROMAS FOR SLEEP

Both ancient customs and modern wellness techniques have a history of using calming fragrances to encourage sounder sleep. The application of aromatic plant extracts for therapeutic purposes, known as aromatherapy, uses the power of different essential oils to create a calming and relaxing atmosphere that promotes sound sleep. Famous for their relaxing qualities are popular scents like lavender, chamomile, and jasmine. These smells function by stimulating the limbic system of the brain, which is important for controlling emotions and mood.

ESTABLISHING A SLEEP-INDUCING AMBIENCE

Creating a sleep-inducing environment is not only about adding nice smells; it's about taking a wholehearted approach to the sensory environment. The atmosphere of the sleeping area is crucial in getting the body and mind ready for sleep. A calm atmosphere is enhanced by soft, muted lighting, cozy bedding, and clutter-free surroundings. When aromatherapy is included, the environment becomes a calming fusion of auditory and visual signals that tell the body to relax. Using aromatherapy sachets or diffusers in the bedroom improves the whole sensory experience and creates a calm environment that is ideal for restful sleep.

AROMATHERAPY NIGHTTIME CUSTOMS

Creating aromatherapy-based nighttime routines might be a useful strategy for telling the body when it's time to relax. Maintaining a regular schedule aids in preparing the body and mind for sleep. Diffusing relaxing essential oils, such as bergamot or lavender, before bed, is a common practice. The body uses the process of inhaling these scents as a cue to go into relaxation mode. The ritualistic element of the nighttime routine can also be strengthened by adding aromatherapy to pre-sleep activities like putting on scented lotion or taking a warm bath loaded with essential oils that promote sleep. In addition to encouraging relaxation, these deliberate activities act as a mental and sensory anchor, indicating that the sleep cycle has begun.

Using calming scents to promote sleep is more than just an aromatherapy exercise; it's a whole strategy for establishing a sleep-friendly atmosphere. People can use scents to help them sleep better and wake up feeling more refreshed if they know how aromatherapy affects the limbic system and include it in a nightly routine in a sleep-inducing environment.

CHAPTER NINE

AROMAS TO PROMOTE EMOTIONAL BALANCE

IMPROVEMENT IN MOOD

Thanks to the strong link between olfactory stimuli and emotional reactions, aromas have a major impact on mood elevation. Certain aromas, such as those of citrus, lavender, and peppermint, have been linked to feelings of optimism.

These scents can release neurotransmitters like dopamine and serotonin when inhaled, which can enhance pleasure and well-being. This phenomenon is frequently associated with the brain's limbic system, which controls memories and emotions.

People who interact with scents that uplift their mood may notice a beneficial change in their emotional state, making mood enhancement natural and non-invasive.

Aromatherapy addresses the complex relationship between smell and the limbic system, which is known to have the ability to balance emotions. Essential oils with relaxing and stabilizing qualities, such as rose, bergamot, and chamomile, are well-known for assisting people in achieving emotional balance.

These scents can promote emotional resilience, lower stress levels, and provide a sense of calmness when inhaled. Aromatherapy for emotional balance entails establishing a peaceful atmosphere in which the selected fragrances complement one another to enhance emotional health.

This all-encompassing strategy for emotional equilibrium emphasizes how crucial it is to incorporate scents into everyday activities to promote mental and emotional well-being.

USING AROMATHERAPY TO SUPPORT EMOTIONS

A therapy technique called aroma inhalation uses scent's ability to uplift emotions. Inhaling particular scents, whether through diffusers, inhalers, or topical application, can directly affect mental health. For example, inhaling essential oils such as lavender or chamomile has been linked to relaxation and a decrease in stress.

With the use of this technique, people can design rituals that are specifically tailored to their requirements and preferences for emotional support. By creating a link between aroma and a feeling of emotional stability, aroma inhalation not only affects one's immediate emotional states but also helps develop a proactive attitude to emotional well-being.

The notions of mood enhancement, emotional balance, and scent inhalation for emotional support are interrelated in the context of aromatherapy.

Through knowledge of the physiological and psychological reactions to particular fragrances, people can use aromatherapy to enhance their emotional health. The integration of these techniques into daily routines can enable a more comprehensive approach to mental and emotional well-being by highlighting the significance of utilizing scents thoughtfully to create intentional and supportive surroundings.

CHAPTER TEN

INCLUDING AROMATHERAPY IN EVERYDAY LIVING

USING AROMATHERAPY AT WORK

Aromatherapy has the potential to greatly improve both employee well-being and the general mood of the workplace. An atmosphere that is calmer and more concentrated can be created in the workplace by using essential oils.

To create a relaxing atmosphere, employers may want to consider diffusing essential oils like chamomile or lavender, which are known for their ability to relieve tension. As an alternative, energizing fragrances like peppermint or citrus can be utilized to increase focus and energy.

In addition to assisting with stress relief, aromatherapy in the workplace promotes a happy and productive environment, which may enhance overall job satisfaction.

Aromatherapy is a lovely method to create a calming and cozy environment in your house. There are several different approaches that one can try, such as utilizing scented candles, essential oil diffusers, or just a few drops of essential oil added to a pot of simmering water. Aromas like tea tree oil or eucalyptus can help create a clean, fresh feeling in living areas. Calm aromas like lavender or chamomile can improve relaxation and the quality of sleep in bedrooms.

Making custom blends according to particular tastes also enables a customized fragrance experience that complements the distinct ambiance of a person's house.

CARRYING AROMA SOLUTIONS ON THE GO

Including portable scent solutions in daily life can be a game-changer for people who are always on the go. Roll-on applicators or personal inhalers that are loaded with essential oils offer a handy method to benefit from aromatherapy all day long. Aromas that are calming, like frankincense or bergamot, can be especially helpful when things get stressful, such as on a busy commute or during a busy day.

These small solutions enable people to discreetly and quickly unwind whenever needed by allowing them to carry their favorite fragrances in a pocket or purse. When looking for a flexible and mobile approach to aromatherapy, portable scent solutions are a great option because of their accessibility and versatility.

Incorporating aroma inhalation into daily life necessitates giving careful thought to the spaces where people spend the majority of their time. Aromatic activities at home create a unique haven for relaxation, while aromatherapy in the workplace can enhance worker productivity and well-being. The versatility provided by portable aroma solutions guarantees that anyone, anywhere, at any time, can benefit from aromatherapy.

CHAPTER ELEVEN

STUDIES AND RESEARCH ON AROMATHERAPY INHALATION

RESEARCH STUDIES IN SCIENCE

Numerous scientific researches have examined the possible advantages of aromatherapy, also known as scent inhalation therapy, for improving both physical and mental health. Scholars have explored the physiological and psychological ramifications of breathing in essential oils, scrutinizing how volatile substances engage with the olfactory system and influence diverse physiological processes. To assure the validity of their results, these investigations frequently use exacting techniques including double-blind testing and randomized controlled trials.

Scholarly inquiries have explored the precise methods by which fragrance inhalation therapy functions. Research has looked into the function of olfactory receptors in the nasal cavity, the neurological networks that carry olfactory signals to the brain, and how this results in the release of hormones and neurotransmitters. This scientific investigation advances our knowledge of the complex relationships that exist between the sense of smell and the body's reaction.

EVIDENCE-BASED APPROACHES

Evidence-based methods are becoming more and more important in the field of aroma inhalation therapy as practitioners and academics work to provide a strong framework for using essential oils therapeutically. Research findings are incorporated into therapeutic decision-making as part of evidence-based practices in aromatherapy, guaranteeing that treatments are not only grounded in custom but also backed by empirical data.

This method strengthens scent inhalation therapy's legitimacy and acceptance in the larger medical community.

Certain essential oils and their chemical components have been found through research to have medicinal qualities, including antibacterial, analgesic, anxiolytic, and anti-inflammatory actions. Based on this information, regimens for aroma inhalation can be customized to address a range of health issues, such as pain management, anxiety, stress, and sleep disturbances. Practitioners can adjust their methods and suggestions in light of the growing amount of knowledge, ensuring that they are in line with the most efficient and proven uses of aromatherapy.

PROSPECTIVE COURSES

There are exciting opportunities for further research and development in the field of fragrance inhalation treatment. A growing number of researchers are concentrating on customized aromatherapy methods, taking into account individual differences in olfactory sensitivity and preferences. As healthcare becomes more individualized, cutting-edge tools like genetic analysis and sensory evaluations may be used to customize aromatherapy treatments to meet each person's specific needs.

Moreover, there is a growing trend toward the incorporation of fragrance inhalation therapy into standard medical procedures. To ensure the safe and efficient use of essential oils in clinical settings, aromatherapists, medical experts, and researchers are working together to establish standardized standards. Aroma inhalation therapy may be included in treatment programs for a variety of ailments as a result of this interdisciplinary approach, which would supplement conventional medical procedures.

Research on aroma inhalation therapy is still in progress and will hopefully offer light on its workings and potential uses in medicine. The incorporation of aromatherapy into healthcare is being shaped by evidence-based procedures, which are also increasing its potential advantages and giving it credibility.

CHAPTER TWELVE

WARNINGS AND RESTRICTIONS

ALLERGIES AND SENSITIVITIES

In a variety of situations, it's important to recognize and manage allergies and sensitivities, particularly when thinking about therapeutic interventions like aromatherapy. Some people may react hypersensitively to particular aromatic compounds or essential oils. Allergies can cause breathing problems, skin rashes, itching, or redness. Before implementing aromatherapy into a wellness routine, practitioners and consumers must be aware of potential allergies and perform rigorous examinations.

Practitioners should obtain thorough medical histories from clients, paying particular attention to any known allergies or sensitivities, to reduce the possibility of unpleasant responses. Patch testing is a useful technique for spotting possible skin allergy responses. Practitioners also need to be aware of the chemical makeup of essential oils because structurally related substances can have cross-sensitivity. Reduce the likelihood of unfavorable outcomes by diluting essential oils and choosing ones with a lesser potential for allergies.

PREGNANCY AND AROMATHERAPY

Because essential oils may have effects on both the developing baby and the expectant mother, the relationship between aromatherapy and pregnancy needs to be carefully considered. Certain essential oils are known to be safe to use while pregnant, but others could be dangerous and should be avoided. It's common advice for expectant mothers to speak with medical specialists before beginning an aromatherapy regimen.

Due to their historical link to uterine stimulation, several essential oils—like jasmine and clary sage—should be used with caution, particularly in the first trimester.

Aromatherapy interventions should be modified by the changing physiological state of pregnant clients, as recognized by practitioners. It is important to take into account individual differences in reaction because certain pregnant women may be more sensitive to specific smells or may feel more queasy as a result of scents.

INTERACTION WITH MEDICATION

There is a chance that aromatherapy will interact with different medications. It is important to know about these interactions to make sure both therapeutic modalities are safe and effective. By influencing cytochrome P450 enzymes in the liver, essential oils can affect drug metabolism and potentially change the pharmacokinetics of prescription drugs. Certain oils can either stimulate or inhibit these enzymes, which can change how much of the medicine is in the blood.

To spot such interactions, practitioners should be well-versed in the pharmacological characteristics of both prescribed drugs and essential oils. It is critical to be transparent with customers regarding the medications they are taking at the moment and to seek advice from medical professionals if needed. People who take drugs with limited therapeutic ranges or are more likely to experience drug interactions should exercise extra caution. Working together, aromatherapists and medical professionals can create treatment programs that are safe, effective, and low risk of side effects.

CHAPTER THIRTEEN

MAKING CUSTOMIZED FRAGRANCE COMBINATIONS

RECOGNIZING INDIVIDUAL PREFERENCES

Understanding individual tastes in great detail is the first step in creating customized fragrance blends. Due to their extremely subjective nature, scents can elicit different feelings and memories in each person. A person's liking for certain smells can be greatly influenced by a variety of factors, including personal associations, cultural background, and early experiences.

It's important to take into account the wide range of fragrances that appeal to different people because what one person finds appealing may turn someone else off. An expert scent maker can create blends that are intensely individualized and appealing to the senses, all while exploring the subtleties of individual preferences.

TAILORING MIXES TO INDIVIDUALS

The craft of creating custom aroma blends entails customizing fragrances to fit each person's unique demands and features. This customization explores the particulars of a person's lifestyle, personality, and well-being in addition to the general, one-size-fits-all approach. Someone looking for energy and focus, for example, would find invigoration in a combination with citrus and peppermint overtones, while someone seeking relaxation and stress relief might benefit from a blend with relaxing lavender and chamomile notes. The secret is to combine different essential oils in a way that complements each person's tastes and objectives, creating a custom scent blend that is as distinctive as the person for whom it is intended.

CASE STUDIES

Analyzing case studies yields insightful information about the real-world implementation of customized scent blends.

These actual cases demonstrate how well fragrances may be customized to fit particular requirements and tastes. For example, a case study can demonstrate how a personalized mix assisted someone leading a busy lifestyle in reducing stress and enhancing the quality of their sleep. A different case study might examine how aromatherapy improves focus and output in the workplace. Examining these examples might reveal trends, triumphs, and difficulties in the process of making custom fragrance concoctions. These studies provide a concrete example of the beneficial effects that customized fragrances can have on an individual's well-being, which inspires and guides aroma designers.

The craft of crafting customized scent combinations centers on a thorough comprehension of human inclinations, painstaking adaptation for each person, and an examination of actual case studies.